IMAGINE LIVING

WITHOUT TYPE 2

DIABETES

IMAGINE LIVING

WITHOUT TYPE 2

DIABETES

Discover a natural alternative to pharmaceuticals.

Dr. J. Murray Hockings, D.C., D.PSc.

Advantage®

Published by Advantage, Charleston, South Carolina.

Member of Advantage Media Group.

ADVANTAGE is a registered trademark and the Advantage colophon is a trademark of Advantage Media Group, Inc.

Printed in the United States of America.

ISBN: 978-159932-495-1
LCCN: 2014932930

This publication is designed to provide accurate and authoritative information in regard to the subject matter covered. It is sold with the understanding that the publisher is not engaged in rendering legal, accounting, or other professional services. If legal advice or other expert assistance is required, the services of a competent professional person should be sought.

For permission to include brief quotations or excerpts from *Imagine Living without Diabetes*, contact the author at:

Help Your Diabetes
3333 Lee Parkway, Suite 600
Dallas, Texas 75219
800-321-9054

Advantage Media Group is proud to be a part of the Tree Neutral® program. Tree Neutral offsets the number of trees consumed in the production and printing of this book by taking proactive steps such as planting trees in direct proportion to the number of trees used to print books. To learn more about Tree Neutral, please visit **www.treeneutral.com**. To learn more about Advantage's commitment to being a responsible steward of the environment, please visit **www.advantagefamily.com/green**

Advantage Media Group is a publisher of business, self-improvement, and professional development books and online learning. We help entrepreneurs, business leaders, and professionals share their Stories, Passion, and Knowledge to help others Learn & Grow. Do you have a manuscript or book idea that you would like us to consider for publishing? Please visit **advantagefamily.com** or call **1.866.775.1696**.

This book is dedicated to the 26 million diabetics, 79 million prediabetics and the millions of families who have lost a loved one to diabetes. My prayer is that this book finds its way into the hands of all diabetics and prediabetics and that they act on this information so they can reverse this terrible disease.

This book is also written in memory of my aunt Lilly, who died of diabetes at the age of 34.

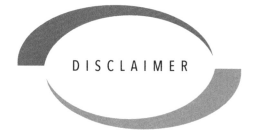

DISCLAIMER

This book is intended for educational purposes only and not for medical treatment of any kind. I am not a medical doctor (thank goodness) and have not been to medical school. However, I do have more than 23 years of experience in natural health care, treating thousands of patients who have been abused by the medical profession (usually unintentionally) and the pharmaceutical industry.

I have been a licensed doctor of chiropractic since 1992 and have been fully trained in nutrition, wellness, exercise, anatomy, physiology, biochemistry, lab interpretation and functional endocrinology.

I am mandated by law to advise you, before you use any of the recommendations in this book, to seek the advice of a licensed medical doctor, even though most have no training in natural health care. This book only contains my opinions from my years of clinical experience and should only be used under direct medical supervision. Before reducing or eliminating any prescribed medications, you should get the advice of your medical physician. None of the recommendations in this book have been approved by the FDA, as the FDA does not approve natural programs but regulates and approves medications. Neither the author, nor any of his subsidiaries, may be held liable for any of the recommendations in this book.

Even though I am protected under the First Amendment of the Constitution of the United States, I am still required to write this disclaimer.

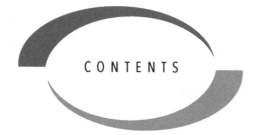

C O N T E N T S

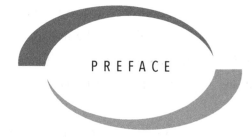

PREFACE

You need to hear the truth.

You are being lied to about diabetes.

Here are the most common lies you are told:

1. Diabetes can't be reversed.

2. Medications are the only things available to "manage" your diabetes.

3. It's a waste of your time and money to attempt to reverse diabetes with natural therapy.

Diabetes *can* be reversed and to say otherwise is a lie. Every month, more and more research is coming out proving that type 2 diabetes can be reversed. UCLA, WebMD, CNN and the Physicians Committee for Responsible Medicine, just to name a few, all say type 2 diabetes can be reversed.

Medications can "manage" your diabetes temporarily, but eventually the meds stop working and more meds are given or higher doses of meds are given until eventually insulin is recommended as a last resort.

Natural therapies are the *only* thing that will reverse your type 2 diabetes—period. Medications will never reverse your type 2 diabetes because they were never designed to reverse it, just to keep you hooked on the meds every day for the rest of your life. This is how pharmaceutical companies become multibillion-dollar empires: by hooking billions of people on medications, not by reversing any disease.

There are other lies, which we will address in this book, but those are the most common.

Why are you being lied to?

There are two main reasons you are being lied to:

1. Money

2. Ignorance

There are three main players responsible for these lies:

1. Pharmaceutical companies (lying for money)

2. Food manufacturers (lying for money)

3. Medical profession (lying from ignorance)

There is no financial incentive for pharmaceutical companies to reverse type 2 diabetes, or any disease for that matter. You need to understand this fact before the rest of this book will make sense. Pharmaceutical companies are multibillion-dollar empires because they don't *reverse* or *cure* disease; they just *treat* and *manage* disease. If everyone on earth were healthy and disease-free, no one would need to take any medications and the pharmaceutical companies would be out of business. If they made drugs that reversed diseases such as diabetes, people would only take the medications temporarily and then get off the meds once they were cured. This also would bankrupt the pharmaceutical companies very quickly.

Now, in their defense, due to the world we live in, medications are sometimes necessary to calm down a crisis or emergency. If you stop taking the medications you are on right now, discontinuing them could have a serious negative effect, perhaps even cause your death. However, once your crisis passes and your blood sugar and A1C (glycated hemoglobin) level is back in the noncrisis zone, you need to take the steps necessary to get your body back in balance so that you can get off your medications. This is not only better for your long-term health; it is common sense.

The food manufacturers who intentionally put ingredients in your foods to make you crave them are also to blame for the lies. The more you crave their foods, the more you buy; the more you eat, the more you crave their foods and the fatter you get, which increases your appetite, which makes you eat more food—and the cycle continues. And while you're getting fatter, eating all the processed, addictive foods, your chance of developing type 2 diabetes increases exponentially. Food manufacturers have no incentive to make non-addictive foods that don't make you fat, because the healthier you are, the less junk food you eat and the less profit they make. It's simple economics 101.

Due to ignorance, the medical profession is the third major player in the lies because medical professionals aren't trained in med school to treat diabetes, or any disease, naturally. They are trained to give you medications or to perform surgery. That's it. So they just tell all their patients what they were taught in school, which is that type 2 diabetes can't be reversed and medications are the only thing available to manage it. I'm convinced they honestly believe that type 2 diabetes can't be reversed. This is explained further in an upcoming chapter, but I truly believe your doctor has no sinister intent when treating you with medications. It's just the way doctors are taught.

What I do have a problem with is when doctors try to make their patients seem foolish for trying to reverse their type 2 diabetes naturally. Many doctors get very negative and defensive when asked about natural options for treating diabetes. Instead of being honest and admitting that they have zero training in natural therapies, they try to talk their patients out of doing something that can help them. This sort of foolish advice reveals their ignorance. If your doctor is against your trying a natural remedy to help you get back in balance so you can reduce or eliminate your medications, you need to fire your doctor and find someone who is open minded on what's best for you. That might seem harsh to you, but your doctor works for you; you don't work for your doctor. There are plenty of doctors where you live and you can find one who is open to your getting healthy naturally. That's the kind of doctor you need on your team.

This book is designed for one reason …

to show you how to get your body back in balance, so your doctor can take you off *all* your medications, because you won't need them anymore.

That is the goal.

Most people can achieve that when they follow the steps in this book and many others can substantially reduce the amount of medications they are taking.

You can do the same thing.

Many people ask me why I have such a passion for diabetes and why my career has led me to focus 100 percent of my time on helping reverse diabetes. It's a very personal reason. My aunt Lily died of diabetes at the young age of 34. It crushed our whole family, especially my uncle Adam (Lily's husband) and their two adopted children, Susan and Brent. I saw her condition progress and eventually lead to cancer, and I felt helpless that I couldn't help her. I was 18 at the time and didn't know what I know now. This heartbreaking story impacted me in a huge way and has led me to my current mission, which is to help prevent type 2 diabetes and reverse it in as many people as possible so they don't have to experience what my family did when Lily died.

The steps in this book are easy to follow, yet they do require some work and you'll have to develop new habits. I'm assuming you don't want to be a type 2 diabetic any longer, which is why you are reading this book. So why not follow the steps inside, reverse your type 2 diabetes, get off your medications and live a long and healthy life? I know you can do it and your family knows you can do it. Yet you won't do it until you make the decision that you *want* to do it.

What are you waiting for? How much worse does your diabetes have to get until you stop messing around and follow the steps in this book to reverse your diabetes? Do you have to start losing your vision, develop neuropathy in your feet, go blind, have some toes amputated? How bad does it have to get? You only get one shot at life, so don't waste another second living with this reversible disease.

I'm on your side and will show you exactly what to do. Are you ready?

It's time to get busy.

DR. J. MURRAY HOCKINGS, D.C., D.PSC.

OCTOBER 2011

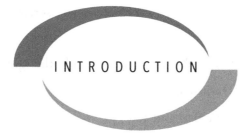

FAMOUS DIABETICS

If you have diabetes, or know someone who does, you're in good company. Many influential people—actors, actresses, athletes, politicians, scientists, business people—are or have been diabetic. Take a look at this list to see just some of the great people who have diabetes:

Adam Morrison, basketball player

Andrew Lloyd Weber, Broadway legend

Anwar Sadat, president of Egypt

Aretha Franklin, singer (who demands your RESPECT)

B. B. King, blues legend

Billy Jean King, tennis player

Carroll O'Connor, Archie in *All in the Family* (1970s)

Dorian Gregory, actor in *Baywatch Nights*

Doug Burns, former Mr. Universe

Elvis Presley, early rock and roll musician

Ernest Hemmingway, author and novelist

Fiorello La Guardia, mayor of New York City

Ghostface Killah, rapper

Halle Berry, actress (Storm in X-men movie series; Catwoman in *Catwoman*)

H. G. Wells, author of *War of the Worlds* and other great tales

Howard Hughes, industrialist

Jackie Gleason, comedian and actor

Jackie Robinson, first African American major league baseball player

James Brown, soul musician

Jerry Garcia, singer and musician in the Grateful Dead band

Johnny Cash, country musician

Kendall Simmons, football player for the Pittsburgh Steelers

Luther Vandross, singer

Mae West, actress

Meatloaf, rock musician and actor (*Rocky Horror Picture Show*)

Mikhail Gorbachev, former leader of the Soviet Union

Mick Fleetwood, rock musician in Fleetwood Mack band

Neil Young, rock singer

Nell Carter, actress

Pam Fernandes, para-Olympian

Paul Cezanne, artist

Piers Anthony, author of fantasy novels (Xanth series)

Ralph Bunche, Nobel Peace Prize winner

Samuel Block, civil rights activist

Scott Coleman, noted for swimming the English Channel

Scott Dunton, famous surfer

Sugar Ray Robinson, boxer

Sylvia Chase, ABC News reporter

Thomas Alva Edison, scientist and inventor of the light bulb

Ty Cobb, baseball legend

Vanessa Williams, first African American Miss America

W. L. Gherra, PayLess drugstore owner

Walt Kelly, cartoonist

Wasim Akram, cricket player

Winnie Mandela, South African politician

Yuri Andropov, leader of Soviet Union

Zippora Karz, soloist in the New York City ballet

TYPE 1

These talented and inspiring people have been diagnosed with type 1 diabetes. Only 10 percent of all diabetics are diagnosed with type 1 diabetes, many of them in their childhood years:

Adam Morrison, National Basketball Association player

Anne Rice, author of the well-known Vampire Chronicles series

Brett Michaels, lead vocalist of the heavy metal rock band Poison

Dorian Gregory, *Soul Train* television show

Gary Hall, Olympic swimmer

Jeanne Smart, actress from television and film (*Designing Women*)

Mary Tyler Moore, actress and present chair of the JDRF

Nick Jonas, singer, Jonas Brothers

Sharon Stone, actress (X-Men movie series)

Sonia Sotomayor, Supreme Court justice, 2009

TYPE 2

Ninety percent of all diabetics are type 2 diabetics. Take a look through this list to see other type 2 diabetics of influence and fame:

Ben Vereen, a triple threat (actor, singer and dancer)

David Wells, a major league baseball pitcher

George Lucas, creator of the Star Wars saga

Larry King, reporter and commentator on CNN

Mike Huckabee, American politician

Patti La Belle, well-known musician from the 1960s

Randy Jackson, cohost, *American Idol*

Sherri Shepherd, cohost, *The View*

CHAPTER 1

WHAT IS DIABETES—REALLY?

At some point in your not-so-distant past, you were likely told that you are a type 2 diabetic or at least that you have metabolic syndrome, which leads to type 2 diabetes. While your doctor was busy telling you that you're going to have to take medications for the rest of your life, that you'll probably have a host of other health problems too, and that you have to watch everything you eat, exercise and lose weight, chances are your doctor didn't take the time to fully explain what diabetes really is, or what causes it, or even how to control it.

So before we go any further, we're going to first explain what type 2 diabetes is.

Simply put, type 2 diabetes is an illness that affects your metabolism. "But what's my metabolism?" you wonder. Your metabolism is the term we use to describe how your body uses food to provide energy and growth for your body. But if something is out of balance—any one of several hormones, for example—you might have an imbalanced metabolism.

When you eat, your body breaks down carbohydrates and transforms them into glucose. In a healthy person, the body produces insulin in the pancreas to help carry the glucose to the cells and to help the cells use the sugars for growth and energy. This reduces the amount of sugar in the blood. If you are a type 2 diabetic, your body becomes insulin resistant. So when glucose is in your bloodstream, it cannot be absorbed by your cells, because the cells aren't letting the insulin bring the glucose into them. The glucose lingers in your blood for some time, and eventually gets released into your urine and out of your body, or gets converted to triglycerides, which is fat.

When your body has really high levels of glucose, the condition is known as *hyperglycemia*. This condition might develop if your body is not producing enough insulin, if your body is not producing any insulin at all, or if the cells of your body have developed "insulin resistance." Insulin resistance is just another way of saying that your cells are not able to properly deal with the insulin that your body does produce. This causes your blood sugar to rise, and your body to "starve," even though there is adequate food to fuel the body.

Diabetes is hardly a new disease or condition. Back in the second century CE, a Greek physician described this condition as *diabainein*. He used it to describe a patient who was drinking and urinating too often. Time passed, languages changed, and eventually, English speakers adopted a Latin variant of the name to describe the same malady.

Over the centuries, a variety of different treatments have been used to deal with this illness. At one time, many were diagnosed for various illnesses, based upon their "humors." This Greek medical system saw the whole body as a collection of "humors" which, when imbalanced, caused illness. By treating the various imbalances, physicians of that time were able to restore their patients to health.

While some methods, especially later, during the Middle Ages and the Renaissance, leave something to be desired, the early Greek physicians got something right. They saw how all the different parts of the body needed to be in balance to stay healthy. They worked with their patients to help them regain their balance and their health.

Now, we don't use the same techniques that the ancient Greeks used, but we do agree with them in principle. We agree that the reason many people are ill nowadays is because their lives are out of balance. They don't eat a balanced diet. They aren't as active as they should be. They don't laugh and cry and express themselves the way they truly need to. They, like you, are out of balance. What we're proposing to do with our Wellness Program is to return your body to a proper state of balance.

Back in classical times, medicine and philosophy were seen as being one and the same. In fact, a lot of our modern medicine has roots in Greek philosophy. Perhaps the best known of the three Greek philosophers who contributed to our modern understanding of medicine is Hippocrates. Many physicians still take the Hippocratic Oath, which was written centuries ago and suggests principles that doctors should live by. In the past, this oath was taken as a solemn promise, something that would have dire personal as well as legal consequences if a physician failed to live by it.

Here is a version of the original Hippocratic Oath, translated into English:

> I swear by Apollo, the healer, Asclepius, Hygieia and Panacea, and I take to witness all the gods, and all the goddesses, to keep according to my ability and my judgment, the following oath and agreement:
>
> - To consider as dear to me as my parents him who taught me this art; to live in common with him and, if necessary, to share my goods with him; to look upon

his children as my own brothers, and to teach them this art.

- I will prescribe regimens for the good of my patients according to my ability and my judgment, and never do harm to anyone.

- I will not give a lethal drug to anyone if I am asked, nor will I advise such a plan; and similarly, I will not give a woman a pessary to cause an abortion.

- I will preserve the purity of my life and my arts.

- I will not cut for stone, even for patients in whom the disease is manifest; I will leave this operation to be performed by practitioners, specialists in this art.

- In every house where I come, I will enter only for the good of my patients, keeping myself far from all intentional ill-doing and all seduction, and especially from the pleasures of love with women or with men, be they free or slaves.

- All that may come to my knowledge in the exercise of my profession or in daily commerce with men, which ought not to be spread abroad, I will keep secret and will never reveal.

- If I keep this oath faithfully, may I enjoy my life and practice my art, respected by all men and in all times, but if I swerve from it or violate it, may the reverse be my lot.

One of the more widely used modern versions of this oath was written in 1964 by Dr. Louis Lasagna, former principal of the Sackler School of Graduate Biomedical Science and academic dean of the School of Medicine at Tufts University. His version follows:

I swear to fulfill, to the best of my ability and judgment, this covenant:

- I will respect the hard-won scientific gains of those physicians in whose steps I walk, and gladly share such knowledge as is mine with those who are to follow.

- I will apply, for the benefit of the sick, all measures [that] are required, avoiding those twin traps of overtreatment and therapeutic nihilism.

- I will remember that there is art to medicine as well as science, and that warmth, sympathy, and understanding may outweigh the surgeon's knife or the chemist's drug.

- I will not be ashamed to say "I know not," nor will I fail to call in my colleagues when the skills of another are needed for a patient's recovery.

- I will respect the privacy of my patients, for their problems are not disclosed to me that the world may know. Most especially must I tread with care in matters of life and death. If it is given to me to save a life, all thanks. But it may also be within my power to take a life; this awesome responsibility must be faced with great humbleness and awareness of my own frailty. Above all, I must not play at God.

- I will remember that I do not treat a fever chart, a cancerous growth, but a sick human being, whose illness may affect the person's family and economic stability. My responsibility includes these related problems if I am to care adequately for the sick.

- I will prevent disease whenever I can, for prevention is preferable to cure.

- I will remember that I remain a member of society with special obligations to all my fellow human beings, those who are sound of mind and body as well as the infirm.

- If I do not violate this oath, may I enjoy life and art, respected while I live and remembered with affection thereafter. May I always act so as to preserve the finest traditions of my calling and may I long experience the joy of healing those who seek my help. (Source: *Wikipedia*)

Nowadays, the Hippocratic Oath is under attack, some claiming that its concepts are archaic and out of place in our modern world. But we at Help Your Diabetes continue to strive toward balance and help our patients reach their best balance so that they can be healthy the rest of their lives without having to take medicines that can kill them, or require them to undergo surgery.

We don't think that concepts such as metabolic balance are outdated or unrelated to living now. We see how the concept of maintaining balance is applicable more than ever, given how busy our lives have become here in North America. That's why we developed this Wellness Program, to help our patients take control of their health and become more in balance.

Insofar as your regular (allopathic medicine) physician is concerned, diabetes is a common, yet chronic, medical condition, which has no cure. As a result, many physicians develop the attitude that the condition can only be "managed" and made more comfortable with drugs to ease the pain or to control other problems that are directly or indirectly a result of having diabetes.

We take a different approach. We know that there are three types of diabetes: type 1, type 2 and gestational diabetes. As far as the Wellness Program is concerned, we are not offering this program for those who have gestational diabetes (which will correct itself after the pregnancy is over), or for those who have type 1 diabetes. *Our Wellness Program is specifically designed with the type 2 diabetic in mind.*

Again, the Wellness Program that we've developed is *strictly for type 2 diabetics.* Why only type 2 diabetics? Why not type 1 as well? It has to do with the specifics of the condition within each type. Let's review what each type of diabetes is really all about.

GENERAL INFORMATION ABOUT DIABETES

According to statistics obtained from the American Diabetes Association, currently, 26 million Americans have been diagnosed with diabetes and it is estimated that 79 million Americans have prediabetic symptoms and conditions at the time of this analysis.

79 million prediabetic Americans. That's a stunning figure, given that our nation's population is around 311 million. This number of prediabetics means that more than one sixth of our nation's population is prediabetic or has what is known as metabolic syndrome. Diabetes is an epidemic. This isn't a virus we're dealing with. It's a way of living that we have chosen that makes us more susceptible to this condition. It comes from the lifestyle that we, as Americans, take for granted. We're always "go, go, go," and our food is heavily processed so that we can keep right on going from one place to another.

Many prediabetics and type 2 diabetics don't realize they have diabetes until they go for a full physical examination with their doctor. The reason for this is simple: there are many symptoms that seem unrelated but are related to the illness. The sooner you are diagnosed with diabetes, the better your chance to avoid serious complications. Without early identification and treatment, you may be more at risk for developing cardiovascular disease, hypoglycemia, kidney failure, retinal damage, ketoacidosis, erectile dysfunction, gangrene, nerve damage and even amputation of the feet. That being said, there are many symptoms that may point to diabetes. By taking the time to explore this list of symptoms, you might be able to prescreen yourself for diabetes. However, the truest test of diabetes is a simple blood test to check your blood glucose levels and A1C, so your physician might determine if you really do have diabetes.

I was diagnosed with Type 2 Diabetes before coming to see Dr. Hockings. I was taking Metformin three times a day, Actos along with other blood pressure medicine, and weighed about 340 lbs. My health was getting bad...After four months of being on the program, I have lost 58 lbs. As I lost weight, my doctor gradually lowered my medications. I started feeling good and now, I don't take any medications at all. I feel 100 precent better. I breathe a lot better. My energy level is high. My doctor can't believe the difference. I have taken my life in control. I would recommend this to anybody that thinks that they're going no-where and feel that their health is in bad shape. It's an easy program, easy steps. I was a non-believer at first because I thought I would never get over it, but in just the short months that I've been in this, it's made a world of difference. After going through this program, I really feel that this program was a life-saver—this saved my life. I feel on top of the world now."

Carl Vann

COMMON SYMPTOMS OF DIABETES

- Consuming more liquids than usual. Are you always feeling thirsty, no matter what and how often you drink? This could be a sign that you have diabetes or at least metabolic syndrome.

- Urinating more often. This symptom goes hand-in-hand with the symptom above, and makes sense if it was simply that. However, when you have high levels of glucose in your bloodstream and you have too little or no insulin to prompt your liver to store that glucose in the fat or muscle cells of your body, your kidney will remove water from your blood (which dilutes the concentration of glucose), which gives you the urge to "go."

- Fatigue occurs when there is inadequate, or no, insulin supply for the body to process the glucose in the bloodstream to fuel the body. This is often in partnership with symptoms of irritability, again due to a lack of energy, as well as intense hunger as your body literally feels it is being starved. This, in turn, can also cause weight gain.

- Those with type 1 diabetes typically describe symptoms of unusual and unexpected weight loss. This is because your body thinks it is starving, so it breaks down fat and muscle tissues for quick energy use. Type 1 diabetes, by the way, tends to set in rapidly, whereas type 2 sets in gradually.

- One thing you might notice is how your extremities (your hands and feet) sometimes feel tingly or numb. This occurs when there is too much sugar in your body, and the crystals of glucose create tiny cuts in your blood vessels. Likewise, this can occur in the eye and cause blurred vision. This also might manifest as a problem with itchy skin, having small cuts and bruises that take a long time to heal, as well as swollen, red gums, gum infection and gum disease.

- Because of the higher levels of sugar in the bloodstream, women may be more prone to vaginal yeast and bladder infections. Both men and women can become prone to other digestive ailments that affect the balance of intestinal flora. And men can develop erectile dysfunction as a symptom of diabetes.

As you can see, diabetes is a condition that affects every part of the body in some way or another. When one part is out of balance, so is the rest. So, if you see yourself in the symptoms described above, it would be in your best interest to visit your doctor and rule out whether you have diabetes or not.

A lot of information about diabetes is available online. A lot of information is also available through the American Diabetic Association. What your doctor will tell you is that your condition is a life-long condition and there is no cure.

But doctors' understanding of diabetes is limited to what they learned in medical school and what pharmaceutical companies give them to treat and manage diabetes. They don't know diabetes the way that I know diabetes. In the next section, I'm going to share with you important information about both types of diabetes to help you understand it the way I do.

TYPE 1 DIABETES

Only ten percent of those diagnosed with diabetes every year are diagnosed with type 1. This form of diabetes tends to be diagnosed in the childhood years or early teens, although it is not unusual for it to be undetected until almost the age of thirty.

What often happens with type 1 diabetes, sometimes called juvenile diabetes, is that the body can't make insulin, which normally helps the body reduce the amount of sugar in the blood. The reason why this happens is unknown. Doctors have been trying to figure out why a previously healthy body suddenly stops producing insulin. It isn't caused by eating too much sugar or being overweight. What they have determined, however, is that the immune system attacks and destroys the pancreas cells that produce insulin. Why the immune system does this, however, is uncertain. Scientists believe that type 1 diabetes is caused by a combination of, perhaps, a person's genetic predispositions and exposure to viruses. Some scientific circles theorize that type 1 diabetes is an autoimmune disorder.

Type 1 diabetes is a serious, chronic disease. The only way for type 1 diabetics to survive is by injecting insulin several times a day, which they can administer themselves or which, depending on the severity of their condition, may require an insulin pump. There are no pills. Because type 1 diabetes is caused by a breakdown of that part of the pancreas that produces insulin, there is *no known cure* for type 1 diabetes. Those who are diagnosed with type 1 diabetes, typically, have a life span that is approximately 15 years shorter than the life span of those who do not have the disease, and type 1 diabetics often experience a lower quality of life as well. This is tragic because most of the people who are diagnosed with this disease are children!

CHARACTERISTICS OF TYPE 1 DIABETES

Typically, someone who has type 1 diabetes reports symptoms such as constant hunger, increased thirst, weight loss, frequent urination, extreme fatigue, and sometimes, blurred vision. If the condition goes undiagnosed and untreated for an extended period of time, the type 1 diabetic can slip into a coma and die.

In extreme cases, and in situations in which DKA (diabetic keto-acidosis) is occurring, type 1 diabetics may also have symptoms such as dry skin and mouth, a fruity breath odor, deep rapid breathing, a flushed face and stomach pain and nausea or vomiting.

It's difficult to keep glucose and insulin levels in the blood regulated, and those diagnosed with type 1 diabetes must check their glucose levels several times a day. This can be particularly challenging with children, as many things impact on the glucose levels. Blood sugar can rise and fall dramatically when there are changes going on. It can vary when children are growing, when people go through hormonal changes, modify their levels of physical activity, develop another illness or infection or change medications. Blood sugar can vary when moods and emotional states change rapidly or extremely, and it can vary depending on what foods are eaten during the day.

Injecting insulin may not always be enough to prevent a hypoglycemic or hyperglycemic reaction, which can be fatal.

Often, when people are diagnosed with type 1 diabetes, they are required to spend time in the hospital until their condition stabilizes. This is mostly because this condition does not attract medical attention until the patient is admitted to hospital in a diabetic coma. A type 1 diabetic must make frequent visits to the doctor to ensure that blood sugar levels are healthy and to learn how to properly conduct blood testing and urine testing at home. This includes being taught how to eat and when, as well as an examination of the food diary (everything you consumed) and your medication diary (times you took insulin).

TYPE 2 DIABETES

When your body does not "properly" use the insulin it makes, you are said to be a type 2 diabetic. Unlike type 1, which is predominantly an autoimmune condition, type 2 diabetes is a progressive condition that takes time to develop. It can still last your entire lifetime, and as time progresses, it may be challenging to keep blood sugar levels within your target range. More than 90 percent of all diabetics are type 2 diabetics and most are overweight. Some are morbidly obese.

Just as in type 1 diabetes, high glucose levels can cause all sorts of problems: blindness, kidney problems, heart disease, nerve damage and erectile dysfunction, to name a few. But by taking care of your diabetes and being a partner in your own health, you can prevent these complications from occurring or delay their onset. Generally speaking, type 2 diabetes is what we call a "40-year-old's disease." By this, we mean that this disease is caused by 40 years of poor decisions regarding food, activity and stress. These poor decisions lead to a variety of interrelated conditions.

With type 2 diabetes, the body becomes resistant to insulin. This type of diabetes can often be managed through weight loss, exercising, or oral medications. However, some type 2 diabetics may still need daily insulin injections.

Type 2 diabetes is considered part of a group of disorders relating to the metabolic system. These disorders include insulin resistance, cholesterol and lipid disorders, obesity, high blood pressure, high risk of blood clotting, and disturbed blood flow to organs. Because of the many interrelated complications from type 2 diabetes, a type 2 diabetic can expect to have a life span that is 5–10 years shorter than that of a healthy person.

Experts suggest that type 2 diabetes progresses in this way:

Insulin resistance comes first. Although your body produces insulin in normal or high levels, it develops a resistance to processing the insulin-bonded glucose and using it effectively.

After a while, the pancreas cannot keep up with the constant demand for more and more insulin. This inability results in a condition known as postprandial hyperglycemia, which causes an abnormal rise in blood sugar after a meal, which can be very dangerous.

Finally, the high levels of glucose in the bloodstream cause damage to the cells within the pancreas, which is responsible for insulin production. This causes the body to stop producing insulin completely, resulting in diabetes.

Generally speaking, some of the complications that a type 2 diabetic can expect are:

- *Damage to small blood vessels*—poor blood circulation in small blood vessels, leading to eye disease, kidney disease, and periodontal disease

- *Damage to large blood vessels*—poor blood circulation in large blood vessels, leading to cardiovascular disease, cerebrovascular disease, stroke and lower limb amputation

- *Nervous system disease*—foot infections and ulceration, decreased sensation, increased sensitivity, muscle wasting, and sexual dysfunction

- *Eye disease*—glaucoma, cataracts and blindness

THE BIG PLAYER IN THIS GAME: YOUR PANCREAS

When you eat your food every day, your pancreas is hard at work. This gland, situated just behind your stomach, is a real enigma. It produces both endocrine and exocrine secretions, which help to control the levels of glucose in your blood—and therefore your body. The two major endocrine secretions that we are concerned with in this book are glucagon, which increases glucose in the blood, and insulin, which decreases glucose levels in the blood. These secretions are produced in the part of the pancreas called the islets of Langerhans, and are critical to the balance of glucose in the metabolism of glucose and its concentration in the bloodstream.

Without insulin, the cells of your body (particularly liver, fat and muscle tissues) cannot absorb adequate amounts of glucose from the bloodstream. When this glucose stays in the bloodstream instead of being absorbed, it can cause a lot of damage to various other organs: the eyes, heart, blood vessels, kidneys and nerves. It can even be fatal.

The pancreas also produces pancreatic fluid, which helps break down the foods that we eat. Fats (lipids), proteins and carbohydrates are made into a chemical soup (chyme) with the help of these digestive enzymes, which enter the small intestine. When these secretions are out of balance, your body faces dire problems as it tries to provide the fuel you need.

WHY GLUCOSE IN THE BLOODSTREAM IS BAD FOR YOU

Glucose is important for the body. Carried through the bloodstream, glucose provides the fuel to keep the body moving. When there is just enough glucose in your blood to fuel your body, it's said that you're within your "target range." But too much or too little glucose in the bloodstream is problematic. Too little glucose in your bloodstream (hypoglycemia) robs you of the energy you need to function properly. Too much glucose in your bloodstream (hyperglycemia) can do a lot of damage to your body if it is not corrected.

Everything you eat is broken down by the body and turned into sugars. Healthy people might be able to eat a donut and feel just fine. But diabetics' bodies are out of balance. So when diabetics eat too much sugar, they put themselves at risk of developing a host of health problems. They can dramatically increase their risk of developing kidney disease, nerve and vision problems, stroke and heart disease.

Signs that you might have high blood sugar:

- *Frequent urination*—When you have high blood sugar, the kidneys work overtime in an effort to flush the surplus glucose out through your urine.

- *Thirst*—When you have high blood sugar, and you are going to the bathroom frequently, you also feel the need to drink a lot. Depending on your beverage of choice (such as soft drinks, for example), you may be making the problem worse.

- *Unexplainable weight loss*—Insulin makes it possible for the cells of your body to use the glucose for fuel. However, when insulin production is low, your body will use stored fat and muscle to feed your cells, which causes weight loss.

- *Fatigue*—When insulin levels are low, the cells in your body cannot get the fuel they need to work, so they don't function well. You often feel tired and unable to take on tasks that you used to enjoy.

DKA AND YOU

We talked about DKA (diabetic ketoacidosis) in the last chapter in connection with type 1 diabetes. DKA occurs when the body doesn't produce enough insulin to allow the cells of your body to absorb the glucose in your blood. At this point, your body starts to break down stored fat, and releases ketones into the blood. Like the unused glucose, these ketones are passed out of your body through your urine.

When there are high levels of ketones in the blood, the blood becomes acidic, which puts your body into an imbalanced state. DKA, if left untreated, can be fatal. However, it is definitely treatable.

SIGNS OF DKA

Extreme fatigue, extreme thirst, frequent urination, dry mouth and other dehydration signs such as a lack of tears are signs of DKA. Without treatment, the symptoms can worsen and can cause pain in the abdominal area, vomiting or nausea, a breath odor that smells like fruit, and deep and rapid breathing.

CONSEQUENCES OF EATING TOO MUCH SUGAR

All your life you have enjoyed sweets and treats and candies. You've thought that they were the perfect thing to end your day, to give you a pick-me-up in the middle of the afternoon or even mid-morning. When you regularly consume high quantities of sugar, particularly refined sugars, you end up doing yourself a lot of harm.

Let's take a look at what happens when you eat sugar-laden products. Given that your body is only really equipped to handle ten to twenty grams of sugar at a time, let's see what might happen if you go to a birthday party. Let's say you don't have any soda or chips, or a hotdog or burger and you are really great about only eating from the vegetable platter and fresh fruits. But that one slice of cake is just too tempting to resist. While you're still smiling from the sweet flavor and the rich texture of the cake, your body begins to react to what you have just consumed: more than *100 grams of sugar* in just one sitting.

Let's see what happens inside you. That sugar hits your stomach and is turned into chyme and suddenly, your pancreas recognizes that there's a ton of glucose in your bloodstream. It goes into emergency production of insulin so that your body can capture that glucose floating through your bloodstream and fuel your body. In the meantime, you feel light-headed, perhaps dizzy. Your nerves are supersensitive. You might feel a bit nauseous. Your heart starts beating rapidly, making you feel flushed or you may feel "high." All this has happened within less than 20 minutes of taking that last bite of cake.

In just a little while, the extra insulin in your body helps your body store that extra glucose by storing some in the muscles and if there isn't any room there, it stores it in your fat cells as—you guessed it—more fat, called triglyceride! You can probably feel yourself getting heavier just sitting there.

Your body is still in shock. It took this massive glucose rush as being a crisis, which created a stress reaction. When your body is stressed, your fight-or-flight instinct is activated, which produces split-second reactions. These stress reactions also make your body release epinephrine (adrenaline) as well as cortisol from your adrenal glands. These hormones (adrenaline and cortisol) stimulate your heart, which begins to race. You feel sweaty, and your mood swings from happy-go-lucky to irritable and stressed in a split second. The cortisol also raises your blood sugar further.

Your body can only take so much stress. Once your body has used up or put away all the excess glucose, there is none left in your blood stream. You run out of energy and you crash. Your body feels as if it's just had its wires stripped. You sit like a lump of dough on the couch. You can't think straight. It's as if your brain has become a blue screen on your computer monitor.

Now, your body's response to that extra sugar was to produce, first, insulin and then cortisol and adrenalin, which did more than just stimulate your stress reactions. When you are stressed, your immune system also takes a hit. Your blood thickens, and some of the cells built to protect your immune system are also damaged. This effect on your immune system can last as little as five hours or much more after eating that slice of cake. In fact, that slice of cake is responsible for making your heart beat faster than normal for another 24 hours. That slice of cake also compromises your immune system for up to 24 hours, making you more susceptible to any virus or bacteria you might come in contact with.

Think you're done with the side effects of that piece of cake? Not even close. Besides having all these hormonal effects, eating too much sugar has other effects that you don't necessarily think about all that much.

First and foremost is dental health. While we know that we *should* brush our teeth after every meal or snack and before bedtime, let's be honest. Very few of us actually do this, unless we are dentists or dental assistants or just plain neurotic. Consuming a lot of sugar is harmful to our teeth, as it makes them decay faster. Failing to keep our mouth clean following ingestion of sugar also can lead to gum disease, which can lead to inflammation of the coronary artery! (Who knew?)

When you eat too much sugar, your body goes on a virtual roller-coaster ride, without the fun. You go on a real high and then drop low, caused by fluctuations in blood sugar, which makes you feel tired. You might also experience headaches or mood swings. While you might eat more sugar to combat the fatigue and other symptoms, the more you do so, the more your body demands sugar to, supposedly, put you back into what it perceives as a normal balance.

When you eat too much sugar, you also become malnourished. You might remember how your parents told you to save the sweets for after your meals. Well, this was for good reason! When you eat sweets before your meal, your body believes that it is full. You see, sugar gives your body a feeling of satisfaction, and makes feelings of hunger disappear. So, rather than eating foods that are more nutritious, you end up eating less of the nutrients you need (iron, magnesium, calcium, and other vitamins and minerals). Additionally—and we all know this by now—when you eat too much sugar, it becomes stored in the body as fat, which can lead to obesity, which can trigger various health conditions such as diabetes and heart disease. Additionally, especially when you consume processed sugars, your body becomes unable to regulate sugar levels because of the processing that the sugar has undergone. For one thing, processed sugar contains little or no chromium, which appears in some unrefined sugars and helps you manage your blood sugar level.

Those who consume a lot of sugars also tend to have an imbalanced immune system. Your body is host to a number of innocuous and beneficial bacteria and yeasts in your digestive system and in your bloodstream. However, when you have a lot of sugar in your bloodstream, the bacteria and yeasts that eat sugar multiply rapidly. This frequent, rapid growth of bacteria and yeast can compromise the health of your immune system, making you more susceptible to illness.

Too much sugar also makes you age prematurely. The process is called *glycation* and what it means is that sugars "stick" to proteins in your body causing the tissues to lose elasticity—not just your skin but also your internal organs—which causes you to age faster. Sugar is also responsible for making it hard for your brain to learn and recognize things. Feeding your children those "chocolate-frosted sugar bombs" before school is a sure-fire way to make sure that they can't remember a thing they've been taught in school. Munching on that chocolate bar or donut before the staff meeting is a sure-fire way to turn your brain to mush when you need it most.

So, now you know what's so bad about sugar and how high blood sugar impacts your health. It's as if sugar literally attacks your body, poisoning you.

Next, let's look at why, although you take all these drugs, you're still not getting better.

"I was kind of skeptical...I knew my blood sugars needed to be taken care of. When I first came in, I had tried a bunch of other things before

... And they worked. I've lost a bunch of weight. My blood sugars are normal. The medical professional gives you pills and tells you to watch what you eat. But you don't know what's good and what's bad. This program makes it easy. This directs you in what to eat and how to eat and it drops your blood sugars. I feel great. I haven't been on medications for three and a half months."

Steve Panter

WHY YOU'RE NOT GETTING BETTER

Many people ask us, given the high cost of their medication, why they aren't getting better. You would think, after spending hundreds of dollars per month on a variety of medications, that you would stop dealing with diabetes and that you would be cured of your condition forever.

However, the sad fact of the matter is that medication that you're mortgaging your house to pay for is not designed to cure you; it is used to "control" and "manage" your diabetes. This method of treating diabetes does not take you into account. It doesn't care about you; it doesn't really want to cure you at all. All it wants is to make money off you and your disease.

Multinational drug companies don't care about you. They sure don't want you to be cured of your condition or you might stop using their products. Their main reason to exist is *not* to cure your problem; it is to earn money for their stockholders. Many businesses make you dependent on their product to supposedly solve your problem. They need you to purchase their product over and over and over again, generating "residual income" for their businesses to continue to thrive. They need you to keep taking drugs every day for the rest of your life to manage your health issues. Every day that you take their drugs, these drug manufacturers make more money. Every day that you continue to let them just manage your health is more money in their pockets and less in yours. These massive corporations are the most profitable corporations in the United States and in the world.

Now, in the USA, we have this regulatory body called the Food and Drug Administration (FDA). The FDA is charged with ensuring that food products and medical products meet certain standards and that the public receives adequate notice of potential harm from consuming these foods or medical products. The problem is this: the FDA can only protect us so far. Unless clinical studies performed on a drug show all the results, including the unpleasant ones, the FDA takes the drug manufacturer's word for truth regarding the safety of the product.

In essence, the FDA is in bed with the drug manufacturers. A high percentage of the members of the FDA advisory panel own stock in the drug companies for which they approve drugs. Yet the FDA does not consider this to be a conflict of interest. The FDA is a self-governing body with no agency overseeing it and that leads to more corruption. Needless to say, this is not in your best interest.

Not that long ago, the FDA gave the drug Avandia (also known as thiazolidinediones or glitazone) a nod and allowed it to be sold in the United States. This medication, used to treat type 2 diabetes, helps to lower blood sugar levels in patients. However, it can also cause fluid retention and sometimes heart failure.

One cardiologist, Dr. Steven Nissen, conducted 42 studies, in which he determined that people who took Avandia to treat their type 2 diabetes were at increased risk of heart attacks by as much as 43 percent compared to people who were not taking any drugs at all. One senator, Charles Grassley, claimed that as many as 100,000 heart attacks may be linked to use of Avandia (stated in the Senate, May 24, 2007).

Avandia was sold to more than 6 million people worldwide, generating 2.2 billion dollars in sales in the USA in one year. Avandia, which ranges in cost from $90 to $170 per month, has been the cause of death for many diabetics. Diabetics, as you know, are already at greater risk of having heart problems than those who do not have diabetes.

In May 2011 the FDA, after serious consideration, announced that, beginning in November 2011, Avandia would no longer be sold in retail pharmacies due to the severity of health risks that it posed to patients. However, this drug is still available through mail order from certified pharmacies that are taking part in a special FDA-supported program. Ironically, this drug, which is killing so many Americans, has been taken off the shelves in many other countries including Germany, the United Kingdom and Canada.

Despite the concerns of many, the FDA approved this drug and allowed it to be sold in the USA. Other forms of the medicine, Avandamet and Avandaryl, are also currently being phased out.

There are more than 26 million Americans who have type 2 diabetes. Almost 500,000 Americans filled prescriptions for rosiglitazone (Avandia) and its sister products in the first 10 months of 2010. After the report came out that Avandia was linked to increased risk of heart problems and heart attacks, the sales of this product dropped dramatically.

Currently, there is a huge class-action lawsuit against the manufacturer, GlaxoSmithKline. How many people are involved? Hundreds of thousands of people are taking up arms and filing class-action lawsuits against the drug manufacturer that put their lives and the lives of their loved ones at unnecessary risk.

After the FDA banned the sale of Avandia, a new drug, Actos, came on the market. This drug became the new "problem-solver" for those who have type 2 diabetes. However, Actos is related to Avandia. It too is a glitazone. On the other hand, it seems to be better than Avandia. According to a study that was published in the *British Medical Journal*, Actos users had 23 percent less risk of requiring hospitalization for congestive heart failure than Avandia users, as well as a 14 percent lower risk of death from any other drug-induced disease. The risk of heart attack was about the same in both groups. The report stated that "switching 1 million patients from Avandia to Actos would prevent 3,700 deaths and 8,300 people from going to hospital."

Named Actos (pioglitzone) in the USA, Glustin in Europe, Glizone and Pioz in India, Actos was the tenth best-selling drug in the USA in 2008, with sales exceeding 2.4 billion dollars. Now Actos is being withdrawn from the safe list of drugs due to increased risk of bladder tumors. The drug is also being withdrawn from markets in countries such as Canada and England, and is being blamed for the untimely death of many who suffer from diabetes and diabetes-related illnesses. Just as with the whole Avandia situation, more and more people are filing class-action lawsuits against the Actos manufacturer.

As you can see, these multinational drug manufacturers only have one interest: getting you to purchase their product so that they can make money. Can you trust them to act in your best interest? No!

You would like to think that your doctor truly has your best interests at heart. And for the most part, many doctors are concerned about providing the best care that they can for their patients. However, they are very busy trying to treat all their patients. Sadly, many patients wait until it's too late before they go to see their doctor with their health concerns. They wait until they have those chest pains, they can't walk very far, feel dizzy and tired, and are having problems breathing before they talk to their doctor about their health.

And doctors who see these patients who wait too long can't do too much to help them. They try to help, but after years of trying to inform and educate their patients about how to live and how to eat, they figure that their patients should know it by now. By the time their patients come to them with a serious condition, they figure that it's already too late and that the only thing left is to medicate them so they can have some level of function and not feel too much pain.

This is what doctors do who have to deal with more and more patients who are diagnosed with diabetes. They have been taught that diabetes is a lifelong condition and they believe that they're doing the right thing for their patients by prescribing medicines that control the illness and related conditions.

The thing is this: Doctors are human. They are not gods. They sometimes make mistakes. They can also be manipulated by pharmaceutical corporations and can fall prey to those representatives who claim that their product is superior to another product. They believe the hype that a pharmaceutical company representative gives them about a medication. While they will most likely read the contraindications, they might miss the fact that certain medications might cause worse problems for their patients than they already have.

You see, pharmaceutical companies have a symbiotic relationship with many medical doctors in the USA and around the world. They leave product samples that doctors, at their own discretion, give to their patients for the condition that the pharmaceutical representative says the product treats. Sometimes this relationship comes with strings attached, and physicians need to provide clinical testing results to the company in exchange for free medicine for patients who cannot afford the drug. Sometimes the sample makes it possible for the doctor to immediately begin treating a client who cannot afford the drug or who cannot obtain the drug right away because the pharmacy is closed, or because of other problems with obtaining the drug.

Some doctors are pressured by drug representatives to offer particular drugs to their patients. They are given bonuses to promote certain products to increase the bottom line of those manufacturers. The more that doctor prescribes of that particular drug, the more money that doctor stands to pocket. We're not saying that all doctors are unethical, but we are saying that doctors are just as gullible as the FDA for trusting drug manufacturers to have patients' health issues at the heart of their business.

Doctors are simply not trained in wellness, clinical nutrition, exercise and prevention. They are trained in diagnosis, treating with medications or treating with surgery. That's all. The difference between what a doctor knows about natural health and what we know is the difference between a dentist and an optometrist. We specialize in natural health, wellness, nutrition, exercise and prevention of illness.

Do you wonder why your doctor tells you to watch what you eat, lose some weight and exercise, yet never explains how to do these three things? Simple: it's because he or she isn't trained in how to do it. He or she is trained to manage chronic diseases, such as diabetes, with medications.

Another reason your doctor thinks diabetes isn't reversible is that he or she has never seen it reversed, which makes sense, as the medications your doctor prescribes for diabetes are not designed to reverse diabetes, just manage it. Day after day, month after month and year after year, doctors see their diabetic patients getting worse, which only reinforces their belief that diabetes isn't reversible.

We're not saying not to trust your doctor. As we said before, your doctor is committed to helping you live a healthy life. What we are saying, however, is that your regular physician has failed you in a very basic way. He or she has failed to teach you and give you the information that you need to make yourself healthy again without use of drugs. Your doctor hasn't provided you with the tools to fix the problem, only the tools to manage the problem. The only way that you, as a health-care consumer, can fully take charge of your health and manage your diabetes is to get off the medication entirely. When you can stop having to use insulin or any other drugs to manage your diabetes and other health complications caused by diabetes, you can protect yourself from the further risk of the deadly side effects of taking these drugs.

I was on nine medications for diabetes, high blood pressure…I was not very healthy and not very happy and hurt all over all the time…I was looking for an alternative to gastric bypass, which my regular physician and my endocrinologist were pushing for me…My mother saw the ad in the newspaper…we decided to try it…I have lost a total of 90 lbs. and I am going to try for my next 50 lbs. in five months. I'm still off all my medications except my high blood pressure medicine now.

Denise Ryan

CHAPTER 3

WHY DIABETICS DEVELOP OTHER CONDITIONS

Most of our diabetic patients have high blood pressure, high cholesterol or high triglycerides. And a high percentage have all three of these dangerous conditions. You probably have one of these conditions too. Have you ever wondered why diabetics typically all have one or more of these three conditions? Has your doctor explained to you why this happens?

If you're like 100 percent of our patients, the answer is no. I've never seen a primary care physician or endocrinologist ever explain why this happens to their patients, yet they will prescribe high blood pressure, high cholesterol or high triglyceride medication. Let us explain to you why diabetics typically get these conditions.

When you have too much glucose in your blood, your pancreas has to release insulin to attempt to bring it down. When you have insulin resistance, which most type 2s have, the glucose can't get into the cells, so it stays in the bloodstream.

High amounts of glucose in combination with insulin act like broken glass in your arteries and cause microtearing in the artery walls. Imagine rubbing sand paper on your face; it's just like that.

These microtears trigger your body to release more cholesterol, which helps repair the microtears in your arteries but then leads to cholesterol build-up, or plaque. Plaque then starts shrinking the openings in your arteries, which increases your blood pressure. The unused glucose converts to triglycerides, which increases fat in your body, which aggravates your diabetes and heart. It's a dangerous domino effect that, once begun, is hard to reverse.

In addition to all these heart complications, many diabetics also have problems with their circulatory and nervous systems, which become damaged by these microscopic tears that occur with the insulin and glucose crystals coursing through their system. These sugary crystals are also responsible for damaging fine nerve endings, such as those to be found in your eyes. Many diabetics, as a result, have impaired vision. Some suffer from some form of diabetes-related eye problem. This can manifest as blurred vision, glaucoma or even blindness.

Some of these circulatory problems begin fairly innocuously. They might start with tingling in the toes or fingers. And while this symptom alone is hardly one to panic about, if you consider that incidences of diabetes are rising in our fast-food nation, consider the consequences of not taking note. Often, one of the early symptoms of diabetes is tingling in the extremities. Once again, this is related to the presence of those shards of sugar crystals coursing through your body, damaging the fine blood vessels in your extremities, including your toes and fingertips. Failure to recognize this as a possible sign of diabetes and having it investigated and making corrections to your eating and lifestyle habits could lead to gangrene and loss of a limb. Why would you do that to yourself? It just doesn't make sense.

What doctors don't talk about are the other ailments that are associated with the disease. They don't tell you about the increased risk of liver failure or kidney failure because of your diabetes. Why not? Because they don't know how to treat your problem until you have it and then they help you to manage it with medication that simply makes the pain more tolerable rather than correcting the problem before it happens.

Your physician knows that once you are diagnosed with diabetes, you have a 70 percent increased risk of dying from heart disease simply because you have diabetes. Again, doctors are simply not trained in wellness, clinical nutrition, exercise and prevention. They are trained in diagnosis, treating you with medications or treating you with surgery. That's all they are trained in.

But it doesn't have to be that way. It isn't impossible to reverse your type 2 diabetes.

The only way to combat this condition is to reduce the level of glucose in the bloodstream, which will, in turn, decrease the level of insulin in the blood, and that will stop the microscopic tearing in the arteries, which will decrease the production of cholesterol, which will open up the blood vessels and arteries and reduce your blood pressure and reduce your triglycerides.

But how do you do this? How do you reduce the glucose levels in your bloodstream effectively? How do you prevent your body from constantly having to respond to some crisis with your blood sugar? Part of the solution is something that is so simple, so easy to do, that you will wonder why you never did it before.

The simple part of the solution is learning what to eat, when to eat it, and how to eat it. Now, there are many eating guides for diabetics. The American Diabetes Association provides a resource book that provides the glycemic index for almost every food. And your regular physician tells you, while prescribing your medication, to watch what you eat. You can buy tons of great cookbooks for diabetics, but none of these resources tell you what you truly need to know.

You need to know *what to eat*, what foods are good for you to eat, and what foods you need to avoid altogether.

You need to know *when to eat*. You need to know how to make sure you have adequate glucose in your system to sustain you all day long. You need to know how many meals you need, and whether you can have snacks or not.

You need to know *how to eat*. In the past, you've eaten tons of processed, prepared foods. You've eaten your vegetables dripping in sauce or cream. You've covered your starch in loads of fat and butters and gravies. You need to learn how to prepare your food so that it is flavorful yet retains its nutrients to give your body everything you need. You need to learn how to order when you eat out so that you don't feel trapped, having to cook all your meals at home every day.

Then you have a hope of being able to control your glucose levels and stay drug-free and healthy for the rest of your life.

The not-so-simple part of combating your diabetes is knowing what supplements or herbs you need to take in order to make your body healthier and help normalize your lab readings.

Having normal-looking lab work after getting your blood tested at your doctor's office is pretty easy with modern medicine. The medications you are taking are supposed to make your labs look normal. However, if you have to take medications to make your labs look normal, you aren't healthy, and you are still a clinical diabetic.

Your goal should be to become clinically nondiabetic: your A1C and blood sugar should be normal without taking any medications. That's where a wellness doctor can help you. Just eating the right way isn't enough for most type 2 diabetics to become clinically nondiabetic. You typically have to take the proper supplements or herbs for a period of time to heal yourself completely. Once your body is clinically nondiabetic, you can, typically, get off most of the supplements and herbs you had to take to be healed, but you will still need to eat the right way for the rest of your life to maintain a clinically nondiabetic state.

CHAPTER 4

THE FOUR ORGANS THAT CONTROL BLOOD SUGAR

When we present seminars about diabetes, we always ask the audience if they can name the four parts of their body that control blood sugar. More than 95 percent of the time, a room full of diabetic patients can't name those four parts. Can you?

If you said "the pancreas, the liver, the thyroid and the adrenal glands," give yourself a hand. However, many people, not just diabetics, don't understand what a fantastic thing the body is, and how beautifully it works together to keep us healthy. When all of these parts are functioning properly, we are healthy. However, when one of these parts is malfunctioning, or has been damaged because of something else we do, the body becomes out of balance.

As we said before, many physicians and endocrinologists don't take the time to explain to their patients how the body works and how their systems are out of balance. If you take a bit of time to learn how the body is supposed to work, you then have some hope of understanding how your body *should* work, and how you are able to return it to a state of balance.

In fact, if you had taken basic biology in school, you might have learned this information. But we're going to assume you never took biology in school, or that you forgot what you learned and that you never learned about how your body functions and how your body is such an amazing organism that works so perfectly when everything is in balance. At worst, this is your first foray into learning about the physiology of the human body. At best, this review will help you revisit what you learned long ago.

THE HUMAN BODY–WHAT A GREAT SYSTEM!

When you learn about the human body, you learn about the different systems of the body. The nervous system sends electrical impulses throughout the body to cause muscles, organs and other components of the body to move and act. The vascular system pumps blood and nutrients throughout your body to bring fuel to the cells and remove waste. The pulmonary system brings oxygen-rich air into the body, through the lungs, into the vascular system, and then to all parts of the body through the blood. It also releases the carbon-heavy waste into the air with every breath. You've studied the basics of the digestive system, in which you have learned how the body takes in food, makes it into a chemical soup, digests it, and expels the waste through urine and feces.

However, there is a system that is often ignored and not taught in high schools, and unless you specialize in it during college, you won't learn anything about it then, either. It's the endocrine system. This system is a very quiet, hidden system that, unless you spend a lot of time learning about hormones, you won't learn about at all. Just as the nervous system sends electrical impulses to muscles, the endocrine system uses hormones to communicate throughout the body.

There are many glands in the body, and each of them produces various chemicals (hormones). Endocrine glands, by nature, don't have ducts, and their hormones are secreted directly into the bloodstream. These hormones act just like messengers and travel through the bloodstream until they reach a specific target organ. When a specific hormone reaches its target organ, the hormone receptors in that organ recognize that hormone and act in a certain way. In many instances, hormones come in pairs, which can turn certain organ functions on or off, speed them up or slow them down, or create a particular response.

THE PANCREAS

Let's review what we talked about in Chapter one. As you remember, the pancreas is the biggest player when it comes to controlling blood sugar. However, it is a big part of your digestive system: it not only breaks down the food in your stomach and turns it into chyme; it is responsible for the production of two hormones that control blood sugar. These two hormones, when working properly, are symbiotic. They balance each other out.

But, like a broken seesaw, when the pancreas is malfunctioning, your body suffers. The two hormones that control your blood sugar are glucagon and insulin. These hormones are produced in the islets of Langerhans portion of the pancreas, which is just behind the stomach. When a healthy body produces insulin, it binds with glucose and is taken into the cells of your body to be used as energy, and the liver responds by removing the extra glucose from the blood and putting it into storage. On the other hand, if the pancreas produces glucagon, the liver responds by taking those carbohydrates that are in storage (as glycogen, in the liver) and uses them to raise the blood sugar levels so that the body can survive.

So, when everything is in balance, your body is able to cope and you're healthy. However, when your body produces too little insulin, or your body becomes insulin resistant, your blood sugar rises. This problem can pose serious complications on a short-term basis as well as on a long-term basis. This condition is what physicians have diagnosed as diabetes mellitus. A physician would say that someone whose pancreas produces inadequate levels of insulin or no insulin at all is a type 1 diabetic. A person whose body becomes insulin resistant, on the other hand, is what a physician would describe as a type 2 diabetic.

Type 1 diabetics can control their blood sugar by taking insulin shots. Type 2 diabetics, on the other hand, may not need to take insulin at all, but may be able to control their blood sugar levels using diet, exercise, and possibly other medications.

THE LIVER

The liver is another part of the endocrine system. Affected by swinging levels of glucagon and insulin, this organ is the one that these hormones affect the most. Because of the balancing nature of these hormones, whatever messages the liver receives, it acts upon. When all is in order, the liver stores excess glucose in the body, by putting it into storage as glycogen, and uses it when there isn't enough glucose in the bloodstream to fuel what the body needs to do.

However, when the body can't utilize the sugar in the bloodstream due to insulin resistance, and the liver has no more room to store the excess sugar as glycogen, the body continues to circulate blood superladen with sugar throughout the system until it finally stores the sugar in fat cells throughout the body, or flushes it out of the system. This is, typically, what happens when someone is diabetic. This process puts a lot of stress on the liver.

THE THYROID

This small gland, which is situated inside the neck, between your trachea (airway) and your Adam's apple is a very important gland. It produces hormones that control your metabolism. When most people talk about their metabolism, they really don't know what it is. Your metabolism is your body's ability to take food that you consume, break it down, and then either store it as energy or to make it into waste products. The two hormones the thyroid produces and which are responsible for this are called T3 and T4. The thyroid gland helps metabolize sugar in your body. So having excess sugar in your system causes extra stress on your thyroid gland, which can cause it to malfunction.

When the thyroid is out of balance, there may be too many or too few thyroid hormones being produced. Insufficient production of hormones causes a decrease in energy, a slower heart rate, constipation, dry or flaky skin, and a feeling of being cold. At times, this condition causes weight gain and may also cause a goiter to develop. Alternatively, when the thyroid is producing too much thyroid hormone, a fast heart rate, unexplained weight loss, diarrhea, anxiety, and even Grave's disease may be experienced.

The thyroid gland regulates your internal and external body temperature as well as your weight. An important part of having a healthy thyroid means ensuring that you are consuming enough iodine in your diet. One way that you can do this is by eating ocean foods such as tuna and salmon, kelp and shellfish, which are high in iodine. Alternately, you can prevent hyperthyroidism by using small quantities of iodized salt as a part of your diet.

When there is already one organ which is not operating properly (namely your pancreas), oftentimes, other organs will follow suit. As a result, diabetics are more likely than a healthy person to develop thyroid disorders. Typically, women are at greater risk of developing thyroid problems, and those who are diabetic are at even greater risk than diabetic men.

Now, the thyroid, as we said, controls your metabolism. This means that your thyroid may be to blame for symptoms that appear to be caused by diabetes. This can be corrected with proper medication. A faulty thyroid gland can really complicate your determination of whether you're diabetic or not, or how to bring the body back into balance if you have both a problem with your thyroid and your pancreas.

Identifying and treating a thyroid problem may well stabilize blood sugar levels. However, it may take time to be able to properly balance your blood sugar levels and make it safe for you to stop taking medication to control your diabetes.

THE ADRENAL GLANDS

The adrenal glands are closely tied into our blood sugar roller coaster. When there is a problem with your blood sugar falling too low or rising too high, these glands kick into gear. They sit on top of our kidneys, and are made up of two parts: the medulla (which is inside) and the cortex, (which is on the outside). The medulla secretes the hormone epinephrine, which we call adrenaline. The adrenal cortex secretes various corticosteroids, which are essential to life.

Adrenaline is produced as a reaction to things that stress the body such as anger, low blood sugar, fright, and caffeine. Yes, you read that right. Caffeine is a stressor to your body! Your body responds to the presence of adrenaline by opening airways to improve your ability to take in oxygen, and also increases your heart rate and the flow of blood to the muscles.

The adrenal cortex produces a variety of glucocorticoids. Many of us are familiar with cortisone and corticosteroids, which are sometimes prescribed for their anti-inflammatory action in a variety of conditions. Though used medicinally at a much higher dose than what your body produces, this hormone tends to suppress the immune system, leaving those being medicated with the drug more susceptible to infections. Cortisol, one of these glucocorticoids, helps to control blood sugar, to increase the fat and protein that are being burned and to respond to stress such as injury, illness and fever. Mineral-corticoids, on the other hand, regulate blood pressure and blood volume by telling the kidneys how much water and sodium to retain.

Now you can see how interconnected everything is. When your adrenal glands produce a hormone called cortisol, it raises your blood sugar. When your blood sugar gets too high, your pancreas releases insulin to bring it down. When your blood sugar gets too low (hypo-glycemic) your adrenal glands release cortisol to bring it up. Insulin and cortisol are supposed to work synergistically to keep your blood sugar in the normal range.

What happens, though, when your adrenal glands are overstimulated from stress, bad diet and caffeine, and they start producing too much cortisol? Your blood sugar rises. When this happens, your pancreas has to produce more insulin to help counteract the high blood sugar due to the high cortisol, which then causes your insulin and cortisol to start working against each other instead of synergistically. Do you think this is good for your body? As you can imagine, it puts a lot of stress on your body, which further escalates the problem.

We have been practicing for a long time and we have *never* seen a primary care doctor or endocrinologist run an adrenal stress index (ASI) test to determine if a patient's cortisol levels are normal. This has stunned us for years because we know that physicians learn about cortisol in medical school and know what it does in the body.

So our question is: why don't doctors automatically run an ASI test on all their diabetic patients, especially since they know how cortisol increases blood sugar? Don't you think that would be useful information for your doctor to have? We think so!

If your cortisol levels are too high and we give you natural supplements and herbs to bring the levels back down to normal, what happens to your blood sugar level? It goes down. When your blood sugar level goes down, do you need to take as much diabetic medication for your diabetes? Of course not.

But, as we discussed earlier, reducing the quantity and types of medications you take isn't high on your doctor's priority list. It certainly is not high on the pharmaceutical companies list. This is why doctors have never had their patients take an adrenal stress index test and why they never will have them take one.

So there you have it: the four most important organs when it comes to controlling your blood sugar. And, again, until now, your doctor probably hasn't taken the time to explain what each organ does to control your blood sugar and how they can become out of balance.

CHAPTER 5

IS TYPE 2 DIABETES REVERSIBLE?

The answer is, "Yes, absolutely."

However, the sooner that you find out that you have the illness, the sooner that you can start to take charge of your health. The key principle required to reverse diabetes is simple: to live life in balance once more. What does that mean for you?

Stop!

First, you need to stop doing the things that promote diabetes.

1. *Stop* eating fast food, processed food, grains, pasta, potatoes and rice. Stop eating candy, cake, cookies. Stop snacking on junk food, chips, and crackers. Stop eating dairy products. Stop drinking soda and coffee. They all contribute to developing diabetes.

2. *Stop* sitting on your butt doing nothing all day. Stop watching so much television. Stop playing video games. Stop being an armchair athlete.

3. *Stop* worrying about every little thing. Stress can literally kill you. Stop micromanaging everyone and everything in your life. Stop being anxious about silly things that

you can't control. Stop worrying about things that will probably never happen.

When you stop doing something, you must replace the "bad" behavior with "good" behavior. I've seen a bumper sticker that reads, "Mother nature abhors a vacuum." It's so true. If you remove a habit or practice, it is important for you to replace that bad habit or practice with a good habit or practice. Otherwise, you might just go back to doing what you've done before simply because you have not thought of what you need to do to succeed. Old patterns are hard to break.

We help you stop those habits that have put you in the condition where you are now. We help you stop by helping you develop new habits, new patterns. We help you *start* anew.

Start!

1. *Start* eating healthy food, lots of fresh vegetables, fruits, lean meats, nuts, seeds, eggs and beans.

2. *Start* being active again. Start by going for a walk and then just keep going. Ride your bike. Roller blade. Dance. Skate. Ski. Play tennis or golf—whatever you love to do to stay active and have fun.

3. *Start* learning how to prioritize things. Learn when to say no to demands from others. Determine what is really important for you to do and let go of things that hurt you. Find a supportive network to help you continue to heal your body and your mind.

As we were talking about just a moment ago, we know how hard it is to break those old habits, the ones that made you who you are today. As a way to help you while you're in transition, and you're learning how to eat healthy, we put you through a full three-week detoxification program. This helps your body get rid of all that toxic sludge in your bowels, in your blood, and throughout your body. After just a few days, your body will stop craving those carbohydrate-loaded snacks that used to keep you addicted to sugar.

You've tried dieting before in an effort to control your weight, perhaps even in an effort to control your diabetes. A lot of the time, though, what happens is that your body starts to tell you that it's not getting as much sugar as it's used to. That's when the cravings start, and the next thing you know, you're chowing down on this triple-chocolate cake with fudge icing, all by yourself. So the detoxification program makes things easier for you. It helps your body to detoxify your liver, kidneys, intestinal track and blood and also helps your body get used to your healthier life choices quickly.

DANGER OF SUGARS

We covered the dangers of eating too much sugar earlier in the book. Let's recap what happens to your body when you eat too many sugars all at once, or if you maintain a pattern of constant consumption of high quantities of sugars.

As blood sugar rises in the bloodstream, insulin levels rise in order to get your body to absorb that sugar into the system. The body becomes insulin resistant and stores excess sugars into as fat called triglycerides, making you heavier and heavier, causing your heart to have to work harder and harder to circulate the blood in your system. This also places a stress on your lungs, which have to work harder to breathe in and out to get an adequate supply of oxygen to your cells. And your bones end up carrying more weight, which causes them more stress and can aggravate arthritis.

The sugar in your blood becomes like broken glass and starts tearing up the sides of the arteries, which causes microtears and scar tissue, which can lead to other complications. Sugar gives your blood a thicker consistency, making it hard to move through your blood vessels, particularly those that are very small. This causes poor circulation in tiny capillaries such as those in our teeth, gums and feet, leading to neuropathies as well as other conditions, such as high blood pressure, high cholesterol, high triglycerides, and so on.

Processed sugar is an incomplete food. Since it contains absolutely no nutrients such as fats, proteins, minerals, fibers, or enzymes, your body "borrows" nutrients and minerals such as sodium, magnesium, calcium, and potassium from healthy cells and bones to metabolize the sugar. Not surprisingly, those who consume vast quantities of sugar often develop osteoporosis at a far younger age than those who do not consume refined sugars. Also, excess consumption of sugar can cause the blood to become overly acidic, which causes the body to draw even more from its mineral stores to correct the problem. However, if the body is already mineral depleted, it loses its ability to process the sugar. It becomes overloaded with waste products and begins to exhibit symptoms of carbonic poisoning.

Also, consumption of processed sugar has been tied to mental problems and depression. Because sugar is an incomplete food, the body must also give up its B vitamins, which are very important to our reaction to stress and maintaining a happy frame of mind. Vitamin B is also linked to healthy production of insulin. Without it, the body is compromised in its ability to manage blood sugar levels.

It's all well and good for us to talk about the dangers of sugar, and how eating too much sugar is harmful to overall health. Part of the key to your success, however, is learning to identify which of the products you regularly consume contain processed sugars. Even if you have been reading the label on the container to see what is in your food, there are many varieties of hidden sugar that you might not know about. According to http://macrobiotics.co.uk/sugar.htm, the average American consumes his or her weight in sugar and more than 20 pounds of corn syrup every year.

That's because many processed foods contain hidden sugars, which makes it tricky for people to accurately track their sugar consumption. This practice of hiding sugars in processed food hurts Americans to the tune of more than 54 million dollars in dental work every year. Most processed food has high levels of both sugars and salts, which make them doubly dangerous for those with diabetes, who are already prone to heart disease and complications.

IDENTIFYING HIDDEN SUGARS

There are many hidden sugars in the food you eat. When you go to the grocery store and pick up a box of crackers, you might be surprised how many types of sugars are hidden within the ingredients list. Sometimes, to confuse you, sugars are listed by other names, by chemical names or by their origin. However, sugar is still sugar and too much hidden sugar could well be your enemy when it comes to regaining control of your health.

Here is a list of more than one hundred "hidden" sugars that you might find if you read the ingredients list on your food package:

Amasake	Glucitol	Microcrystalline cellulose
Apple sugar	Glucoamine	Molasses
Barbados sugar	Gluconolactone	Monoglycerides
Bark sugar	Glucose	Monosaccharides
Barley malt	Glucose polymers	Nectars
Barley malt syrup	Glucose syrup	Neotame
Beet sugar	Glycerides	Pentose
Brown rice syrup	Glycerine	Polydextrose
Brown sugar	Glycerol	Polyglycerides
Cane juice	Glycol	Powdered sugar
Cane sugar	Hexitol	Raisin juice
Caramelized foods	High-fructose corn syrup	Raisin syrup
Carbitol	Honey	Raw sugar
Carmel coloring	Inversol	Ribose rice syrup
Carmel sugars	Invert sugar	Rice malt
Concentrated fruit juice	Isomalt	Rice sugar
Corn sweetener	Karo syrups	Rice sweeteners
Corn syrup	Lactose	Rice syrup solids
Date sugar	Levulose	Saccharides
Dextrin	"Light" sugar	Sorbitol
Dextrose	"Lite" sugar	Sorghum
Diglycerides	Malitol	Sucanat
Disaccharides	Malt dextrin	Sucanet
D-tagalose	Malted barley	Sucrose
Evaporated cane juice	Maltodextrins	Sugar cane
Evaporated cane juice	Maltodextrose	Trisaccharides
Florida crystals	Maltose	Turbinado sugar
Fructooligosaccharides	Malts	Unrefined sugar
(FOS)	Mannitol	White sugar
Fructose	Mannose	Xylitol
Fruit juice concentrate	Maple syrup	Zylose
Galactose		

It is easy to use natural sweeteners, such as stevia, to give yourself that sweet taste without actually adding sugar or harmful chemicals such as aspartame (NutraSweet) and sucralose (Splenda) to your diet.

Now, you can spend hours reading labels and trying to find each and every type of sugar that has been hidden in your food, but the Wellness Program we offer is far easier. Simply by eating whole, unprocessed fruits, vegetables, meats and nuts, you will automatically almost eliminate all those hidden sugars without worry. So you'll get to enjoy lots of nutritious and delicious food without having to try to find out if there are sneaky processed sugars in your food.

Taking supplements can also really help in your goal to heal your body and return it to health and vigor. Some supplements can really impact your ability to absorb certain nutrients. What many people with diabetes and other disorders relating to metabolism don't realize is that they may be horribly malnourished! Well, it only makes sense. If you're getting most of your daily caloric intake from eating sweets and breads and pasta and rice, you're not getting much in terms of nutrition. You're missing out on some important vitamins and minerals that your body needs to be healthy. Amazingly enough, when your body starts to get those vitamins and minerals from your good food choices and from supplements, you become healthier in no time at all. Even better, using the right supplements can quickly get rid of food cravings and also help you feel better, healthier, and more energetic quickly!

Eating proper foods is the key to managing your diabetes. However, it's not enough to just avoid the bad stuff. You need to eat nutrient-dense foods, and then know when to eat them and how to prepare them for maximum benefit. There will be no more cakes, cookies, biscuits, buns, rolls, cereal, or bagels! No more frying, batters, pizza, pasta, white or red potatoes, crackers, or rice! No more milk, cheese, butter, or ice cream! No more soda, chocolate, desserts, coffee, or caffeinated teas either!

Now, before you get all depressed thinking about what you can't eat, there is a long list of things you *can* eat. This short list will give you some idea of what you can eat, but there is so much more!

✓ You can enjoy many delicious fruits: apples, apricots, bananas, bilberries, blueberries, black berries, boysenberries, breadfruit, cantaloupe, carambola (starfruit), cherries, clementines, cranberries, currants, dates, durian, figs, grapes, grapefruits, guava, honeydew, huckleberries, jackfruit, kiwis, kumquats, lemons, limes, loquats, lychees, mangoes, nectarines, oranges (all kinds), papayas, passion fruit, pears, peaches, persimmons, pineapple, plantains, plums, plumcots, pluots, pomegranates, quinces, raspberries, strawberries, tamarinds, ulgi fruit, watermelons, and that's just a start ...

✓ You can fill up on low-calorie and nutrient-rich vegetables: alfalfa sprouts, artichokes, artichoke hearts, arugula, asparagus, avocado, bamboo shoots, bean sprouts, beet greens, beets, bell peppers, bok choy, broccoli, broccoflower, brussels sprouts, cabbage, carrots, cauliflower, celery, Swiss or red chard, chick peas, Chinese cabbage, chives, collard greens, cucumbers, eggplants, endive, garlic, green beans, green onions, green peas, greens, horseradish, jicama, kale, kidney beans, kohlrabi, leeks, red or green or iceberg lettuce, lemon grass, lentils, lima beans, mushrooms, mustard greens, navy beans, okra, onions, peppers, pumpkins, radishes, radicchio, rhubarb, rutabagas, shallots, snow peas, soy beans, spinach, split peas, summer squashes, sweet potatoes and yams, tomatoes (all kinds), turnip greens, turnips, water chestnuts, watercress, winter squashes, zucchinis, and many, many more.

✓ You can get your protein from a variety of sources: abalone, alligator, American bison, anchovies, basa, bass, caribou, cat fish, carp, cattle, chicken, cod, clams, conches, crabs, crayfish, crocodiles, cuttlefish, deer, duck, eel, emu, flounder, geese, goat, groundhog, groupers, grouse, haddock, halibut, hare, herring, lamb, lobster, mackerel, mahi-mahi, marlin, moose, mussels, octopus, opossum, orange roughy, ostrich, oysters, partridge, peccary, perch, pheasant, pigeon, pig, pike, pollock, prawn, quails, rabbit, salmon, sardine, scallop, sheep, shrimp, snails, snapper, sole, squid, tilapia, trout, turkey, tuna, veal and more.

✓ You don't have to stop going out for a coffee break with your friends; you can just switch your beverage choice to a caffeine-free tea, and use almond milk, rice milk, coconut milk, or water for your beverages.

You can substitute grains with quinoa and cream of buckwheat without guilt.

While you're getting your eating habits under control, the next thing to tackle is changing your life and adding exercise to the mix. It's important when you first get started exercising again to do the right kind of exercise. Some people will go and try to lift tons of weight right away. It's important to do the right kind of exercise to help support your goals. If you're like many type 2 diabetics, you're quite heavy, possibly obese. If you have been inactive for a long time, and do something that is too strenuous too soon, you could hurt yourself, and potentially have a heart attack and land in the hospital. This could really be detrimental to your success and could cause you to backtrack or worse.

When you have managed all of these together, your doctor will likely be able to take you off many of your medications that you have needed in the past. Why? Because your body will have started to heal all on its own, and you will become more and more in balance: more alive, energetic, healthy, sexy, strong and happy.

Diabetes can be reversed!

CHAPTER 6

WHAT IS YOUR HEALTH WORTH?

If today, you could place a value on your health, what would you say it's worth? For many of us, this is a really tough question to ask. We're used to thinking about the value of our home, or the value of our car, but how do we determine the value of our health?

Well, try to think of it this way:

Maybe you spend about ten thousand dollars to go on vacation with your family every summer. But right now, you're experiencing full-blown diabetes. You have to take thousands of dollars' worth of drugs every year to manage your diabetes, and other conditions that are exacerbated by diabetes.

The cost of continuing to live the way that you are living now is that you will likely die 5 to 15 years before your healthy, nondiabetic friends will. It is unlikely that you will live to see your grandchildren finish high school or college. You definitely won't make it to seeing your great-grandchildren being born. Is that a price you're willing to pay?

What would it be worth for you to be able to live, healthy and full of energy, for 10 to 15 more years than you would if you continued to live the way you do today?

What would it be worth for you to be able to see your grand-children finish college, get married, and have children of their own?

What would it be worth for you to be able to go on those vacations that you love so much without pain or drugs, and without needing to take frequent breaks because you're just too tired?

Many of our prospective patients say, "I really want to do your program and help reverse my diabetes, but it depends on what your meal plan will be." When we hear this, we can't help but feel confused. Here are people who obviously *want* to change their life, but they have these conditions attached to their desire. These "conditions" are contrary to their achieving their desire. They might say something like:

"I want to get better but I can't give up…

- bread

- rice

- soda

- beer or mixed drinks

- cheese

- ice cream

- coffee…"

and so on.

This mentality is a classic example of unrealistic expectations. These people are looking for a way to have their cake and eat it too—literally. It's because of this way of thinking that many people choose drastic measures, such as bariatric surgery or lap-band surgery, to lose weight, rather than making the lasting changes that will help them live longer and healthier for a long time. These surgeries offer a quick-fix solution, but they do not provide lasting results because, invariably, the patients return to the same patterns that have led them to be the way that they are. The best way to lose weight and to reverse diabetes has been proven, consistently, to be intrinsically tied to learning how and when to eat better foods.

People who have bariatric surgery or lap-band surgery can lose a significant amount of weight very quickly, which in turn can calm down or potentially stop their diabetes, but it is only temporary, because these procedures don't teach them how to think differently about food and how to eat better. They still eat the same junk, just less of it, due to the medical procedure. Almost all those who have undergone the above-mentioned two procedures have their diabetes return full force very quickly. These procedures are short cuts, and should be avoided at all costs.

When deciding whether to participate in a natural Wellness Program, such as the one we offer, you need to decide how important your health is to you. You need to place a value on your health. You need to decide which is more important to you: drinking a soda or being able to see a sunrise; eating cheese or having your feet amputated because of gangrene; eating pasty white bread or dying of a heart attack. It comes down to a decision—your decision.

Every day, thousands of people quit smoking "cold turkey." They think about it for a while, hemming and hawing and talking about it. Maybe their family has been begging them to stop smoking. It doesn't matter, because a smoker will continue to smoke until ready to stop smoking. You can educate smokers about the dangers of smoking and they can just keep right on puffing away in front of you. You might threaten to take away their cigarettes, or to leave them, or you might try bribery to get them to stop smoking. But until smokers make the decision for themselves—a conscious decision that *this is it*—they will continue to smoke.

The American Health Authority recognizes that smoking is a difficult habit to break. The reason it's so hard is because of the addictive nature of nicotine. Its lack causes extreme discomfort for ex-smokers, making them crave the drug so badly that unless they have strong support, a strong will and good medical support as well, they most likely will start smoking again. But making the changes necessary to reverse diabetes is far easier than quitting smoking. All you have to do is change the way you eat, take a few supplements, and exercise a little.

What decision will you make?

Some might say, "I really want to get better, but it depends on how much it costs." And here, again, they are putting their values in the wrong place. Sure, money is important. But without health, what are you going to do with that money?

If the cost of being able to fully reverse your diabetes—to the point that you'd never have to worry about it again for the rest of your life, be off all your medications, get your energy back, get your sex drive back, sleep better and have no doctor visits every couple months—were $10,000 to receive treatment for six months, would you do it? Is your life worth $10,000?

Some patients would say $10,000 is too much. But our question is: "Too much compared to what?" You will easily spend more than $10,000 on cosmetic dentistry for implants or crowns or veneers. You might spend $10,000 on plastic surgery. You can easily spend $10,000 or more for a couple of nice vacations over the next few years. And you will definitely spend more than $10,000 for your car, which only lasts so long and then you have to replace it. Most people are completely happy with spending $10,000 on these things that don't save their life and that don't, ultimately, have any lasting value.

But when people think of their health, they don't see the value of investing in it. They don't see the value of a program that costs $10,000 and allows them to live another 20 years as an investment. Broken down into smaller numbers, that translates into only $500 per year for 20 years, or about $42 per month. You spend more money on buying coffee at the local coffee shop than you do on your health. What good does it do you to keep $10,000 in your pocket if you don't have your health, or if your quality of life won't let you enjoy the money you've saved, or if you die prematurely? Isn't your health worth more than that? The great news is, the Wellness Program we offer is not even close to $10,000. We were just using the $10,000 as an example to see where your head is.

Sadly, many people abuse their bodies. They eat food that has little or no nutritional value. They eat foods that are high in fats and loaded in sugars. They drink lots of beer, wine, or mixed drinks. They work really hard, sometimes at backbreaking jobs, sometimes at superstressful jobs, in an effort to provide for their family and to save some of their money for their retirement. Their dream is to retire and spend the rest of their life relaxing, carefree and doing the things they love.

The thing is this: When they finally retire, they retire with a host of health problems. They're like a ticking time bomb about to go off. They suffer from chronic diabetes. They have high blood pressure. They have heart complications. And instead of spending their retirement years enjoying the good life and their family and friends, they end up spending their saved money on medical care that doesn't make them healthy or keep them healthy.

What is your health worth?

I know for a fact that people who lose their health and are dying in the hospital aren't telling themselves, "I'm sure glad I saved that few thousand dollars and didn't invest in a natural program to get myself better."

Recently, a former palliative caregiver from Australia, named Bronnie Water, blogged (www.inspirationandchai/regrets-of-the-dying.html) about the five most common wishes of the dying. She lists them from one to five, but we're going to reverse them and talk about each of them in turn.

REGRETS OF THE DYING

Number 5: I wish I had let myself be happier. Lesson: Happiness is a choice, and the sooner that we allow ourselves to be happy, and to experience happiness, the sooner that we can share it as well. We don't have to pretend that we're happy with situations that are making us sad. Choose happiness, choose laughter, choose joy.

Number 4: I wish I had stayed in touch with my friends. Lesson: When we're dying, suddenly we want to be close to those who knew us best a long time ago. Our parents are gone (most likely), and having the company of those who "knew us when" makes our final months, weeks, days, and hours meaningful. Love and relationships are the most important things in life. Nurture your friendships your whole life long.

Number 3: I wish I'd had the courage to express my feelings. Lesson: On your deathbed, you don't leave words unsaid that should have been said. The words you should have spoken to your child, your partner, your friend, your enemy—they need to be said. You can't say those words to those who have already passed on. Make peace (if that's what's needed) with those you want to and let go of relationships that are harming you. It's okay to do that.

Number 2: I wish I hadn't worked so hard. Lesson: On your deathbed, you're not going to be so concerned about the workload that you need to do today, tomorrow or next week. You're wishing that you hadn't spent so much time at the office instead of spending time with your family, even if you had only sat at the table for dinner more often, listened when your teenager ranted about a bad day at school, or attended your child's dance recital. Live your life now. Spend time with your family now. You might not have a chance later.

Number 1: I wish I'd had the courage to live a life true to myself, not the life others expected of me. Many times, you might have let someone else tell you who you are and what you should be, instead of living the life that you dream of. Maybe you nurture a secret dream of being a nurse. Maybe you nurture a dream of being a clown. Maybe you nurture a dream of being—anything that you dream. Live your dream while you can.

Bronnie made a point of saying that "from the moment you lose your health, it is too late. Health brings a freedom very few realize, until they no longer have it." Live your dream now, so that you don't regret it when it's your time. Don't let your dying wish be that you wished that you had placed more importance on your health than on your work, the house, the car, or anything else for that matter. *Without your health, you have nothing.* You can't spend more time with your family. You can't go scuba diving at the Great Barrier Reef. You can't go parasailing. You can't climb Everest. You can't even see your grandchildren being born.

What is your health worth?

Less than a century ago, people lived a simpler life. It's true. Cars were just starting to be built. The industrial revolution was in full swing. Trains crisscrossed the country. Planes were an experiment, not a mode of transport. And technology such as electric ranges, refrigerators, televisions, microwave ovens, computers, cell phones, mp3 players and digital readers were things that were yet unimagined. But back then, despite the fact that people worked long, hard hours in the fields, and despite the fact that they ate large meals, people took care of themselves. They went to see the doctor when there was a problem. They took care of their health themselves, as best they could. They didn't have the same kind of pressure that we have now in our society at work. They didn't have processed food, dripping with processed sugars and salts. They ate "whole" food, fresh food, in season. They ate what was available when it was available. And they lived to be 100 years old and over, before passing away, still "sharp as tacks," still active and still healthy, just old and tired.

Now, despite all of our great achievements as a society and the fantastic things we have achieved in the past hundred years, it seems shameful that people are dying younger and younger every year. How many children can say that they know their great-grandparents these days? How many grandparents get a chance to see their grandchildren graduate high school or college? Not too many! It's shameful that these people never get to see their grandchildren marry or to see their great-grandkids being born. People are dying in their 60s and 70s when they should easily live well into their 90s or even past the age of 100. Why are they dying so young? For many, it is diabetes and diabetes-related illnesses.

You can resign yourself to that reality if you want to. You can *choose* to have to live your life with a full medicine cabinet just to treat all your illnesses, and still feel sick and tired and useless. You can choose to never see your grandchildren because you're in the hospital all the time. You can choose to allow yourself to die much younger than you should.

But I don't think that you want that. I think that you want to *choose to live pain-free, drug-free for the rest of your life*. I think that you want to *choose more time with your family and friends*. I think that you want to *choose more laughter and more life* to celebrate with the people that matter to you. I think that you want to *choose to live a long, healthy life*.

And why do I think that? Because you chose to read this book. Because you chose to really think this process through. So now, *the choice is yours*. Choose wisely.

My triglycerides were over 3500—in less than 60 days they were down to 200. My cholesterol was at 564—they fell to 194...I've lost 40 lbs. I'm off of all my medications except for a small asprin.

Richard Mayo

CHAPTER 7

ARE YOU READY–REALLY READY?

What will it take before you decide to take the plunge and make the commitment to change your life for the better? Will it take that first heart attack? Losing your foot? Blurred vision? If you wait for these symptoms to surface before you take action, it may all be too late!

When you're ready to take charge of your health, to be a partner in your own cure, and to choose a longer, healthier life, we're ready to work with you. But don't think this will be an easy thing. We won't lie. It's a challenge.

Our society and culture shape us from our infancy. During our lifetime we learn to eat food that is bad for us and ends up making us sick. We are taught by our families, friends and media to *crave* that burger, those fries and that soft drink. Eating food that is bad for us is addictive. We experience sugar highs and lows based on how much and what we eat. We get incredibly high blood sugar levels when we eat that donut or cake yet feel great when we eat lean protein or a light salad with a tiny bit of dressing. It's not just a physical thing; it is emotional as well.

And eating good food takes a lot of work. It takes becoming educated about your food choices. It means learning how to read the label on the box and how to identify hidden sugars, salts and other nasty things that are hidden in our processed food. It means learning that there is more than just one kind of apple to eat. It means learning how to stop purchasing processed food and how to cook for ourselves. This skill is essential when it comes to learning how to eat healthy instead of eating sugar-laden foods at all your meals.

Our program has been tested time and again. By following our program explicitly, we guarantee that you will achieve remarkable results. You might even be able to stop taking all those medications for your heart, your high blood pressure and diabetes.

We have you start a three-week detoxification for your body. Using a combination of supplements, powdered drinks, and liquids, you continue to eat *real* food—fruits, vegetables and meat. We know how hard it is to stop eating the rich, fatty, carbohydrate-loaded food that is slowly killing you. That's why this detoxification is so important. This is a gentle but thorough cleanse and detoxification. By the time you've done the three weeks, your liver, kidneys and intestinal tract will be cleansed. You'll actually feel better, more energetic and full of life.

Following your cleanse, we will go over the results of your initial laboratory testing and explain in detail what is wrong and how your body is out of balance. At this point, we will recommend various, customized, nutritional supplements and herbs, and provide you with dietary recommendations to help you get your body back in balance. We'll explain to you, simply and easily, what to eat and how to eat so that you can regain control of your health.

While you follow our recommendations, we follow up with you, and continue to encourage you to maintain the work that you have already started. You'll stay on this specialty diet and nutritional supplement and herb regimen for about two to six months, being monitored throughout. At the end of your program, we will conduct another series of tests to evaluate how much you have improved throughout our program. This will help you clearly see the difference between your life before our Wellness Program, and your life after the Wellness Program.

Most of our patients, following our treatment, are able to dramatically reduce the amount of medications that they are taking or are able to stop taking them altogether, because their primary physician agrees that they no longer need them, based on their latest laboratory test results. Our patients experience dramatic but healthy weight loss. They report having greater energy to carry out their tasks during the day, and to spend time with family and friends. They report having more of a sex drive, not to mention feeling sexier and more attractive. They tell us that they sleep better, and feel more refreshed, and are able to think more clearly throughout their day. They feel strong, healthy and—most importantly—most are able to stop taking all their diabetic medications, including insulin, *with their doctor's approval.*

Don't believe these claims? Here are the words of some of our clients:

I have gotten off all my thyroid, diabetes and heart medications.

Jean Munsen

I was having problems with my blood sugar. It was running up as high as 300…when I saw the ad in the paper, I knew I had to do something. I was afraid to go to my medical doctor because I knew that they would put me on insulin and I don't like needles…I have lost 56 lbs. I take no medication. I feel great. There is no comparison. I couldn't sleep at night. I had all kinds of problems ... All that is gone. And it's really hard to believe that it's so easy. All I did was change my way of eating, and the weight just started dropping off; my clothes sizes went down. It's easy to maintain the style of eating too. I haven't had any problems.

Eleanor Adams

Now, we know it's a challenging program. We're not going to lie. But with our support, we can make this promise: if you follow our directions *exactly,* you will succeed in your goal to take your life back. The only thing that might make it fail is you. If you don't follow the program explicitly, you won't get results, and you will likely have to continue taking medication for the rest of your life. Is that what you really want?

You need to choose: life with insulin injections and drugs that can kill you, or *our Wellness Program.*

Changing your life can be really tough all on your own. It's even harder when you're the main cook for your family, or you don't have support from your family members, colleagues or friends. Our Wellness Program provides full support to help you learn how to change your lifestyle so that you can enjoy a long, healthy life.

The program tackles the three lifestyle components that are directly related to diabetes: diet, exercise and stress. Not sure what to eat and when and how much? We tell you what to eat, how to prepare it, and how much to consume. Not sure how to get started exercising again? Not sure what is safe for you? We get you moving again, doing some moderate exercise to get your heart pumping in a good way and improving your cardiovascular health, and we help you reduce stress while you're at it. Finally, we get you to take a few supplements every day to improve your results.

Again, it's *your choice*. You can choose a short, unhealthy life supporting big pharmaceutical companies, or you could *choose right now to change your life for the better, become drug-free and healthy forever.*

CHAPTER 8

CUSTOMIZED PROGRAMS AVAILABLE FOR THOSE WHO QUALIFY

Many diabetics try to get better on their own by following diabetic meal plans, exercising a bit and taking some supplements. However, many never achieve their goal of reversing their diabetes. The biggest reason is that it takes a lot of mental energy and time to always be thinking about what you're eating, and when and how you're going to prepare your food. Professional athletes have a coach who tells them, "You can eat this now, that later, and that later still."

Think of us as your personal food coaches. We'll show you, step by step, what you should be eating and when, in order to reverse your diabetes. We'll show you how much food you need to eat, and what kind of food you need to really fuel your body, to help it remove those years of bad eating and lifestyle habits, and to start being healthy again. With our help, you can be assured that you will succeed in finally getting your diabetes under control.

In order to be accepted in our customized, one-on-one program, you must first qualify to participate.

How do you qualify?

1. You must be 100 percent committed to following our Wellness Program exactly as we instruct.

2. You must be willing to invest in our program.

3. You must stick with it for the whole length of the program and not quit.

We believe that your life is worth living and that it's worthwhile for you to be able to enjoy a long, drug-free, and healthy life. To ensure that you get the full attention of our vigilant team, we only treat a certain number of patients a month. We want to make sure that you get personal, one-on-one attention, whether you choose to sign up with us for a two-month plan or a six-month plan, to help you reverse your diabetes. Our Wellness Plans are specifically developed for the needs and concerns of type 2 diabetics.

With any of our custom plans, you can rest assured that you are getting a great start on bringing your type 2 diabetes under control. We are committed to providing you with accurate and thorough laboratory interpretation to help you reach your goal of reversing your diabetes and being able to live without drugs to control your health.

You begin your program with a full, three-week cleansing and detoxification program. This program helps remove toxins from inside you, safely and effectively, making it possible for you to clean out the harmful sugars that have been accumulating in your body and making you crave more sugar. In just a few short days, you will, typically, lose your interest in eating sweets.

Once you have started on the program and have finished the cleanse and detoxification, and we have given you your results from the laboratory testing, we provide you with your own supply of customized herbs and supplements to deal with your specific issues for the length of your program.

During your program you have one-on-one follow-up by telephone with our team of doctors. You can also enjoy unlimited support from our clinic by e-mail or telephone to answer any questions you might have.

Finally, we provide you with exercise recommendations to help you reverse your diabetes.

We can only accept a limited number of patients each month, due to the high amount of time we spend with each patient, and the high level of customization we give patients for their specific program. To get more information on whether you qualify to be a part of our one-on-one programs, call 800-321-9054.

Now that you've finished reading this book, if you continue to have your type 2 diabetes, it's for one reason …

you are choosing to.

Type 2 diabetes can be reversed. The next step is up to you.

Dr. J. Murray Hockings, D.C., D.PSc.

October 2011

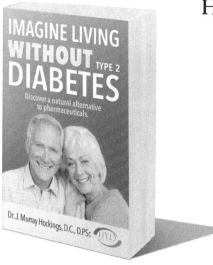

How can you use this book?

MOTIVATE

EDUCATE

THANK

INSPIRE

PROMOTE

CONNECT

Why have a custom version of *Imagine Living without Type 2 Diabetes*?

- Build personal bonds with customers, prospects, employees, donors, and key constituencies
- Develop a long-lasting reminder of your event, milestone, or celebration
- Provide a keepsake that inspires change in behavior and change in lives
- Deliver the ultimate "thank you" gift that remains on coffee tables and bookshelves
- Generate the "wow" factor

Books are thoughtful gifts that provide a genuine sentiment that other promotional items cannot express. They promote employee discussions and interaction, reinforce an event's meaning or location, and they make a lasting impression. Use your book to say "Thank You" and show people that you care.

CPSIA information can be obtained at www.ICGtesting.com
Printed in the USA
LVOW01s1730160415

434880LV00020B/857/P

9 781599 324951